Prenatal Nutrition: The Science and Wisdom of adequate diet for Pregnancy

Dr Sandra P. Martinez

TABLE OF CONTENTS

Chapter 3

WHAT I SHOULD AVOID DURING MY FIRST TRIMESTER?

1. Don't smoke

2. Steer clear of alcohol

3. Steer clear of undercooked or raw meat and eggs

4. Steer clear of sprouts that are still in their raw state

5. Avoid particular seafood

Chapter 4

FOODS THAT HELP A BABY BECOME HEALTHY

Chapter 8

EXERCISE

What types of activities are safe to engage in while pregnant?

Why is exercise healthy for a pregnant woman?

Which workouts ought to be avoided when pregnant?

SUMMARY

Points To note

INTRODUCTION

Maternal nutrition is essential for the health of a mother and her unborn child during pregnancy. Health issues for the woman and her fetus can result from inadequate nutrition during pregnancy, both in quantity and quality. Malnourished mothers are more likely to experience preterm labor, maternal mortality, gestational anemia, hypertension, miscarriages, and fetal deaths during pregnancy. It may result in low birth weight and fetal intrauterine growth retardation in the newborn, which may have long-term effects on the infant's development, quality of life, and medical expenses. The newborn's immune system's development is negatively impacted by malnutrition. Determining the association between maternal nutrition and fetal growth is therefore crucial. Prospective cohort research involving 150 pregnant women was conducted in Menufia Governorate's maternal and child health care facilities. Maternal malnutrition and maternal and infant outcomes were significantly correlated.

Women need to eat healthily and safely before getting pregnant to build up enough reserves. Energy and nutritional requirements rise throughout pregnancy and lactation. In the womb and throughout early childhood, women's health and the health of their kids depend on meeting these needs. However, the nutritional status of women is appallingly inadequate in many regions of the world. Too many women, particularly young people and those who are nutritionally vulnerable, do not receive the nutrition services they require to maintain their health and provide their unborn children the greatest possible chance to live, grow, and develop.

Chapter 1

WHY IT'S IMPORTANT TO EAT WELL WHILE PREGNANT

Why Consume Real Foods While Pregnant?

Real, nutrient-rich, whole meals provide your body with the nutrition it needs to develop a healthy baby. Your baby's health will be at its best if you eat well and store nutrients properly as a mother. Additionally, consuming real foods throughout pregnancy might help prevent anemia and lower your chance of developing pregnancy-related conditions like gestational diabetes, preeclampsia (high blood pressure), and preterm labor. Pregnancy diet optimization also aids in postpartum recovery.

Generally speaking, eating well has a lot of advantages. A healthy diet gives a woman several benefits, including increased stamina, a better immune system, and a lower chance of illness, to name a few. Because they are also eating for the health of their unborn child while they are pregnant, pregnant women need to be extra careful about what they consume. When a pregnant woman eats healthily, she lowers her risk of issues like anemia, low birth weight, and birth abnormalities. Healthy eating might also lessen uncomfortable pregnancy symptoms! The advantages of a good pregnancy diet are listed below.

Mom and Baby Benefit From a Healthy Diet

Less complexity

Although it might be challenging, resisting undesirable pregnancy cravings is ultimately beneficial for the well-being of both you and your unborn child. You can be at risk for issues like gestational diabetes, anemia, urinary tract infections, and the birth of a child with birth abnormalities if you don't follow a balanced diet. It's never a bad thing, but healthy eating throughout pregnancy can help make labour and delivery easier!

Enhanced Energy

For the majority of women, feeling so exhausted during pregnancy that they can barely move is extremely typical. No matter what you do, exhaustion can often be challenging to manage, especially in the first few weeks when your body is going through a lot of hormonal changes. By maintaining an appropriate weight, blood pressure, and blood sugar levels, you can lessen the likelihood of developing such issues. Your energy levels will be maintained by consuming a healthy meal and doing so every 3 to 4 hours. It's vital to keep in mind that your iron needs should be doubled throughout pregnancy to support your larger blood volume and encourage the fetus's ability to store iron.

Positive fetal development

A healthy diet is just what your baby needs to develop properly. You should try to consume at least 300 more calories each day than usual. You don't want to overdo it, either, as that can result in issues like preeclampsia and gestational diabetes. A healthy newborn needs a variety of vitamins and nutrients, including but not limited to calcium, folic acid, vitamin C, vitamin A, fiber, fruits, vegetables, whole grains, and enough protein and fat.

Better Sleep

During your pregnancy, a lot of things can keep you awake at night, including nausea, many toilet trips in the middle of the night, or aches and pains! Your beauty sleep will undoubtedly benefit from eating regular, substantial meals and abstaining from excessive caffeine. Iron, calcium, and vitamin B are among the vitamins and minerals required during pregnancy that also promote restful sleep.

Lower Chance of Being Ill

Pregnant women are more susceptible to contracting certain illnesses, such as the flu. This can be avoided with a balanced diet and lots of sleep. Although a simple cold won't likely harm your unborn child, experiencing pregnancy symptoms is unpleasant enough without adding sickness to the mix. It's best to try to be healthy in general!

Specialists in High-Risk Pregnancy in NJ

Along with eating well while pregnant, you should prioritize receiving the right prenatal care. Every patient at New Jersey Perinatal Associates receives individualized care and is fully informed of all decisions made for their health and the health of their unborn child, thanks to the close collaboration between our perinatologists and our referring physicians. We are delighted to assist women with high-risk pregnancies at every stage since we recognize that the existence of specific risk factors can increase the stress of pregnancy. Find out more about our perinatologists, including their qualifications and areas of specialization:

Decreases the likelihood of birth defects

Birth abnormalities in your child might result from exposure to specific substances or a dietary deficiency. Birth abnormalities like spina bifida are more common and have been related to a shortage of essential nutrients like folic acid. It's essential to eat as many natural, unprocessed foods as you can when pregnant in order to avoid harmful poisons. It is also necessary to take a high-quality prenatal vitamin in order to maintain proper nutrient intake, particularly for critical components like iron and folic acid.

Ensures Your Baby Has a Healthy Weight

Compared to kids delivered at a healthy weight, low birth weight babies experience more health issues and even life-threatening consequences. Low birth weight might predispose infants to lifelong health issues or disabilities. Make sure you're getting enough calories and nutrient-rich foods to help your baby healthily grow weight. During pregnancy, you should consume at least 300 additional calories each day, the majority or all of which should come from wholesome meals such as whole grains and vegetables.

Your baby will not only acquire a taste for foods that are low in nutrients if you eat badly, but he or she will also be more likely to become obese and suffer dangerous conditions like diabetes. However, if you maintain a healthy diet while you're expecting, you'll help your child develop in a way that will benefit them for the rest of their lives. Additionally, you will be promoting your baby's healthy eating practices.

Helps you lose weight more quickly

The majority of women are eager to eliminate any excess pregnancy weight as soon as feasible. In addition to increasing your chances of gaining a healthy amount of weight throughout pregnancy, eating healthfully also makes it simpler for you to lose that weight once you give birth. It will be simpler for you to eat properly and maintain a healthy weight if you practice healthy eating habits during pregnancy and after the birth of your child. You'll also serve as a good example of healthy behavior for your child! It's crucial to maintain a healthy diet when pregnant. Everything you eat affects both your health and the growth and development of your unborn child.

NOTE

Eating well throughout pregnancy gives a woman several benefits, including increased stamina and a better immune system. When a pregnant woman eats healthily, she lowers her risk of issues like anemia, low birth weight, and birth abnormalities. Pregnancy diet optimization also aids in postpartum recovery. Pregnant women are more susceptible to contracting certain illnesses, such as the flu, which can be avoided with a balanced diet and lots of sleep. It's essential to eat as many natural, unprocessed foods as you can when pregnant in order to avoid harmful poisons.

During pregnancy, you should consume at least 300 additional calories each day. Eating healthfully also makes it simpler for you to lose weight once you give birth. You'll also serve as a good example of healthy behavior for your child! It's crucial to maintain a healthy diet when pregnant.

Chapter 2

PRENATAL FOOD NUTRITION

A balanced, healthy diet might also aid in easing certain pregnancy side effects, including nausea and constipation. A daily increase in caloric intake of about 300 calories is required to support a healthy pregnancy. These calories ought to come from a diet rich in protein, vegetables, fruits, and whole grains.

The following foods are beneficial to your health and fetal development during pregnancy:

Protein

Aim for 80 to 100 grams of protein per day from sources like eggs, almonds, avocado, pasture-raised animals and birds, nuts, and whole milk dairy products because they are the basis of life and are essential for your developing kid.

Fat

Did you know that our brains are primarily composed of fat and that vital fatty acids, which we obtain from food, are necessary for all of the brain's structures and functions? Consider including fats from unprocessed natural foods like meat, dairy, and plant-based oils like olive, avocado, and coconut oil. It's best to start building this when your kid is developing. Limit processed vegetable oils that are high in Omega 6 fatty acids, such as corn, soybean, and peanut oil, and try to consume more Omega 3 fatty acids.

Vegetable

The vitamins and antioxidants found in non-starchy veggies are beneficial to you and your unborn kid (such as leafy greens and cruciferous vegetables) and are crucial throughout pregnancy. By cultivating and preserving diverse gut microbiota, they can also reduce constipation.

Suitable Carbohydrates

A high-carb diet during pregnancy, particularly one high in refined carbohydrates, is associated with an increased risk of gestational diabetes, preeclampsia, gallbladder disease during pregnancy, and metabolic issues for the unborn child. It is crucial to choose the proper carbs, which include whole and unprocessed grains, fruits, vegetables, legumes, and full-fat dairy products. Target 100-150 g each day.

Fluids

Water is essential for maintaining healthy circulation, which carries nutrients to your baby, helps with digestion, transports oxygen, controls body temperature, and eliminates waste. Go for 100 ounces per day.

As a side note, I find that eating healthy during the first trimester and the start of the second is quite difficult for me (and many others). Therefore, keep in mind that even during those weeks when all you can stomach is mac n' cheese, cereal, pizza, etc., the meals you ate before becoming pregnant can still keep you nourished.

Chapter 3

WHAT I SHOULD AVOID DURING MY FIRST TRIMESTER?

It's time to get to work as a new mom. Even though you can't prevent every difficulty, you may use these useful suggestions to have a positive, healthy first trimester.

1. Don't smoke

As soon as a woman learns she is pregnant, she should consult her doctor about strategies to give up smoking. A woman shouldn't smoke at any point while she is pregnant. Smoking during pregnancy increases the risk of birth abnormalities in the child. Additionally, because the nicotine in e-cigarettes can harm a developing baby's brain and lungs, they are not safe to use while pregnant.

2. Steer clear of alcohol

No alcohol intake is deemed safe during pregnancy. Drinking during the first trimester can result in birth abnormalities, miscarriage, stillbirth, and fetal alcohol spectrum disorders, which include behavioral and intellectual problems (FASDs)

3. Steer clear of undercooked or raw meat and eggs.

The risk of listeriosis and toxoplasmosis, which can cause serious and life-threatening diseases, severe birth abnormalities, and miscarriage, exists in raw or undercooked meat and eggs.

4. Steer clear of sprouts that are still in their raw state

Salmonella and E. coli are possible contaminants.

5. Avoid particular seafood

Mercury levels in tilefish and mackerel are high.

6. Steer clear of unpasteurized juices and dairy products

Soft cheeses like feta, Brie, and goat cheese are among them.

These might have listeria bacteria in them.

7. Steer clear of processed foods like deli meats and hot dogs

These might also have listeria.

Additionally, nitrates and nitrites are present.

8. Limit your caffeine intake

It's acceptable to consume some caffeine: around 200 mg (2 cups of coffee)

Coffee can alter a baby's heart rate and pass through the placenta.

9. Aim to maintain a healthy weight

The first trimester is not the time for pregnant women to "eat for two" (women usually need more calories during the second and third trimesters, but not necessarily during the first)

Pregnant women who put on too much weight increase the likelihood that their unborn children may develop obesity.

10. Steer clear of steam rooms, hot tubs, whirlpools, and saunas

A pregnant woman visiting these locations runs the risk of hyperthermia, dehydration, and fainting.

Especially in the first trimester, a considerable increase in the mother's core temperature may have an impact on the growth of her unborn child.

According to some studies, using one of these during the first trimester while pregnant may double the risk of miscarriage.

11. Do not get a massage or acupuncture

Although these treatments are generally safe for use throughout pregnancy, the first trimester is not the time to massage a pregnant woman's abdomen.

While acupuncture is generally safe to use while pregnant, several acupuncture points should be avoided.

When receiving acupuncture, ladies should confirm that the practitioner has experience treating expectant mothers.

12. Do not clean your cat's litter box

Toxoplasma gondii, a parasite that is present in cat waste, can result in miscarriage, stillbirth, or major health issues in newborns.

13. Do not use specific cleaning products

Make sure there are no pregnancy warnings on the labels of cleaning products.

Naphthalene, a substance found in several toilet fresheners and mothballs, can harm blood cells.

14. Prevent artificial tans

Although they normally pose no risks when used during pregnancy, they may trigger an allergic reaction.

Pregnancy hormone levels make the skin more sensitive and can increase a woman's susceptibility to allergy responses.

Avoid using tanning supplements or injections.

Chapter 4

FOODS THAT HELP A BABY BECOME HEALTHY

There are a ton of delectable selections that provide you and your infant with everything they'll need. Inform your medical team about your eating habits, and allow them to help you develop a plan that includes any essential supplements.

Dairy products

You must consume more calcium and protein. Throughout pregnancy, to fulfill the demands of your developing fetus. Milk, cheese, and yogurt are examples of dairy items that need to be considered. Casein and whey are two types of high-quality protein that are included in dairy products. Dairy is the best source of calcium and contains large levels of phosphorus, B vitamins, magnesium, and zinc.

Since Greek yogurt contains more calcium than the bulk of other dairy products, it is particularly helpful. Probiotic bacteria, which assist digestive health, are also present in some kinds.

You might be able to handle yogurt, especially probiotic yogurt, if you have lactose intolerance. To find out if you can try it out, ask your doctor. There may be an entire universe of yogurt parfaits, smoothies, and lassis waiting.

Legumes

Lentils are excellent plant-based sources of fiber, protein, iron, folate, and calcium, all of which your body need more of during pregnancy. This food group also contains peas, beans, chickpeas, soybeans, and peanuts (a.k.a. all kinds of amazing recipe ingredients!). One of the most crucial B vitamins is folate (B9). It's crucial for both you and the unborn child, especially in the first trimester and even before. You must consume at least 600 micrograms (mcg) of folate daily, which can be difficult to do through diet alone. However, if your doctor advises supplementation, including legumes can help you get there.

Legumes typically include a lot of fiber. Iron, magnesium, and potassium levels in some kinds are also high. With dishes like hummus on whole grain toast, black beans in a taco salad, or lentil curry, think about including legumes in your diet.

The sweet potato

In addition to being tasty and prepared in a variety of ways, sweet potatoes are also high in beta carotene, a plant chemical that your body converts into vitamin A. Vitamin A is crucial for a baby's growth. Just be careful with animal-based sources of vitamin A that are consumed in large quantities, such as organ meats, as they can be poisonous.

Fortunately, sweet potatoes are a good plant-based source of fiber and beta-carotene. Fiber prolongs satiety, lowers blood sugar surges, and enhances digestive health (which can help if that pregnancy constipation hits).

Try using sweet potatoes as the base for your morning avocado toast for a fantastic breakfast.

Salmon

Salmon is a nice addition to this list, whether it's smoked on a whole wheat bagel, teriyaki-grilled, or covered in pesto. Salmon is full of beneficial omega-3 fatty acids, which are present in high concentrations in fish and help develop the brain and eyes of your unborn child, as well as lengthen gestation. Has someone advised you to consume less seafood because it contains toxins like mercury and other high mercury fish? You can continue to consume fatty fish like salmon.

The following fish should be avoided because they have high levels of mercury.

swordfish

shark

Queen Mackerel

marlin

large-eye tuna

from the Gulf of Mexico, tilefish

Additionally, salmon is one of the few naturally occurring sources of vitamin D, which is deficient in the majority of us. Both the immune system and bone health depend on it.

Eggs

Those amazing, edible eggs are the healthiest food you can eat since they have a small amount of practically every vitamin you require. A big egg has about 80 calories, as well as lots of vitamins, minerals, and high-quality protein and fat. Eggs are also a fantastic source of choline, which is essential for pregnant women. It is crucial for a baby's brain growth and aids in preventing improper brain and spine development. You can get closer to the current advised choline intake of 450 mg per day trusted source while pregnant by consuming one entire egg, which has a choline content of approximately 147 milligrams (mg) (Trusted Source) (though more studies are being done to determine if that is enough). The healthiest ways to prepare eggs are listed below. Try them in a chickpea scramble or spinach feta wraps.

Broccoli and leafy, dark vegetables. It should come as no surprise that broccoli and other dark, green veggies like kale and spinach are incredibly nutrient-dense. They may frequently be snuck into a variety of foods, even if you don't particularly enjoy eating them. Benefits include fiber, vitamin C, vitamin K, vitamin A, calcium, iron, folate, and potassium. They are a veritable treasure trove. Servings of green vegetables are an effective approach to increase vitamin intake and prevent constipation because of all the fiber they contain. Additionally, vegetables have been associated with a lower risk of low birth weight Trusted Source.

You won't even notice that there is kale in this Florentine recipe for kale eggs or a green smoothie if you add some spinach to it.

Lean proteins and meat

Lean meats like chicken, pork, and beef are great sources of high-quality protein. During pregnancy, you'll need more of the B vitamins, choline, iron, and other nutrients found in beef and pig. Iron is a necessary component that red blood cells utilize to make hemoglobin. Your blood volume is increasing, so you'll need extra iron. This is crucial during the third trimester of pregnancy. Iron deficiency anemia may result from low iron levels in the first and second trimesters of pregnancy, which increases the danger of low birth weight and other problems. It may be challenging to meet your iron requirements just through food, particularly if you have a meat allergy or are a vegetarian or vegan. But for those who can, eating lean red meat frequently may help you obtain more iron from your diet. Combining foods high in vitamin C with foods high in iron may aid enhance absorption. Examples of such foods are oranges and bell peppers. Make this steak and mango salad, or top that turkey burger with vitamin-rich tomato slices.

Berries

Berries have a relatively low glycemic index rating, so they shouldn't cause significant blood sugar increases. They also contain water, nutritious carbohydrates, vitamin C, fiber, and antioxidants. They make fantastic snacks because they are high in fiber and water. Some of the greatest berries to consume while pregnant are blueberries, raspberries, goji berries, strawberries, and acai berries. They offer a lot of flavor and nutrition yet have few calories. For some ideas, look at this blueberry smoothie.

Whole Grains

Whole grains have significantly more fiber, vitamins, and plant components than their refined cousins. Instead of white bread, spaghetti, and white rice, consider oats, quinoa, brown rice, wheat berries, and barley.

Oats and quinoa are two examples of healthy grains that also have a decent amount of protein. Additionally, they stimulate other areas that are frequently deficient in pregnant women: B vitamins, fiber, and magnesium.

There are countless ways to include healthy grains into any dish, but we enjoy this quinoa and roasted sweet potato bowl.

Avocados

Because they have a high concentration of monounsaturated fatty acids, avocados are a unique fruit. They are also high in fiber, B vitamins (particularly folate), vitamin K, potassium, copper, vitamin E, and vitamin C. Due to their abundance of healthy fats, folate, and potassium, avocados are a fantastic pregnancy food since they help to maintain blood sugar levels (and always).

Folate may help avoid neural tube defects and developmental disorders of the brain and spine like spina bifida, and healthy fats help build the skin, brain, and tissues of your child.Leg cramps, a common side effect of pregnancy for some women, may be relieved by potassium. In actuality, avocados have a higher potassium content than bananas.

You may use them as guacamole, in salads, smoothies, and on whole wheat bread, as well as mayonnaise or sour cream replacement.

Stale fruit

In general, dried fruit has a lot of calories, fiber, and different vitamins and minerals. One serving of dried fruit can supply a significant portion of the daily requirements for many vitamins and minerals, including folate, iron, and potassium. One serving of dried fruit contains the same amount of nutrients as one piece of fresh fruit, just without all the water and in a much smaller form. Prunes are a good source of potassium, fiber, and vitamin K. They are effective natural laxatives and can aid with constipation. However, dried fruit also includes significant amounts of natural sugar. Dates are high in fiber, potassium, iron, and plant components. Although dried fruit may assist improve calorie and nutrient consumption, it's often not advised to consume more than one serving at a time. Be sure to avoid the candied versions, which contain even more sugar. For a portable snack that is high in protein and fiber, try adding a tiny amount to a trail mix with nuts and seeds.

Salmon liver oil

The oily liver of fish, most frequently cod, is used to make fish liver oil. Supplementing with fish oil may help prevent premature delivery and may aid fetal eye development since it is high in the omega-3 fatty acids EPA and DHA, which are crucial for the development of the fetus's brain and eyes. A lot of individuals don't receive enough vitamin D, and fish liver oil is a great source of it. For people who don't consume seafood frequently or take omega-3 or vitamin D supplements, it might be quite helpful. Fish liver oil contains more omega-3 fatty acids, vitamin D, and vitamin A per serving (1 tablespoon or 15 milliliters). However, it's not advised to consume more than one serving daily because too much-preformed vitamin A can be harmful to your unborn child. Additionally, high omega-3 intake may have blood-thinning effects. You can also achieve your omega-3 goals by eating low mercury seafood such as pollock, sardines, canned light tuna, salmon, and sardines.

Lentils

The B vitamin folate, also known as folic acid in supplements, is abundant in lentils and essential for the development of your baby's brain and nervous system. Spina bifida, a disorder in which the spine does not correctly develop during pregnancy, and other neural-tube defects like it are also strongly inhibited by it. Lentils' high fiber content can keep your digestive system in working order and help you avoid constipation during pregnancy. This vegetarian protein source should be on your menu whether you consume meat or not. Around 7 milligrams of iron and 17 grams of protein are found in a cup of cooked lentils.

And to top it all off, lentils are versatile and simple to prepare.

The Pregnancy Daily Dozen provides all the vitamins, minerals, and nutrients you and your unborn child require in 12 simple food groups. Try firm French or black lentils in salads, use softer brown lentils in place of chickpeas in your favorite hummus recipe, or make a thick, stew-like soup with creamy, fast-cooking red lentils.

Yogurt

Calcium is essential for both you and your baby's growing bones, as well as for healthy nerve and muscle function and strong bones. Your daily calcium requirements can be met with three to four servings of dairy products, with yogurt being one of your finest options. It has the same amount of calcium per cup as milk and is also a good source of protein, iodine, and folate. However, not all yogurts are made equal. Active cultures, or good bacteria, in yogurt can also aid in preventing stomach distress and yeast infections (which are more common in pregnancy). Since plain varieties don't contain any added sugar and are simple to customize with add-ins, they may be preferable to flavored ones. If you'd like, try adding some honey or chopped fresh fruit to it to make it sweeter. In addition to eating yogurt straight out of the cup or bowl, you can also mix it with granola to produce a creamy-crunchy parfait, use it in place of sour cream or mayonnaise in dips, sauces, or baked goods, and add yogurt to smoothies.

Nuts

Speaking of being little but mighty, Along with protein, fiber, and healthy fats, nuts are packed with essential vitamins and minerals like magnesium, zinc, potassium, and vitamin E. They also travel well, making them the perfect pregnant snack. Are some varieties superior to others? All nuts have distinctive nutritional profiles and can be included in a balanced pregnancy diet. However, some might be particularly worthwhile. Almonds and walnuts both contain calcium, and walnuts are particularly high in omega-3 fatty acids. Peanuts, too? They contain a lot of folates. (Who knew?)

Use nuts to add flavorful crunch to oatmeal or yogurt, or grind them and use them in place of breadcrumbs for chicken or fish dishes.

Carrots

Their bright orange color means that carrots are crammed with beta-carotene, which the body converts to vitamin A. And that nutrient is critical for your baby's developing eyes, skin, and organs. In addition to munching on the go, try shredding carrots and folding them into pancakes, muffins, or quick bread batters. Alternately, you may steam them and then mash them like sweet potatoes with a little butter and cinnamon.

Red peppers

In addition to fiber to keep things moving, these vegetables are a high source of vitamins C and A. Another important benefit? According to research, consuming a diet heavy in vegetables may help lower the risk of issues including preeclampsia and high blood pressure.

The next time you have a yearning for chips or pretzels that are crispy, take advantage of their crunchy texture. They make a great snack when dipped into hummus, ranch dressing, or simply plain yogurt.

Kale

The leafy green is always a smart move and is an especially effective superfood during pregnancy. Folate, iron, vitamin C, calcium, vitamin A, vitamin E, vitamin K, and fiber are all provided by kale, which is both pleasant and versatile. Try replacing the basil in your favorite pesto recipe with kale, adding it to spaghetti, building a sandwich with it, or incorporating it into scrambled eggs.

Oats

The 25 to 30 grams of fiber per day that are advised will help you feel fuller for longer and prevent painful pregnant constipation. The good news is that one cup of cooked oats contains more than 4 grams and more than 30% of your recommended daily intake of magnesium, a mineral that is essential for your baby's development of strong bones and teeth. Hot breakfast oatmeal is not your thing? Try substituting oat flour for all-purpose flour in your favorite baked products. Oats may be ground into flour in a food processor.

Bananas

When you feel the want to eat something, anything, right away, they are a tasty source of energy. Additionally, they are comfortable for your stomach even when you are feeling sick. (Vitamin B6 in bananas is connected to reducing morning sickness during pregnancy.) Additionally, bananas contain a lot of potassium, a mineral that is essential for maintaining healthy blood pressure. Since potassium helps your body discharge puff-promoting elements like salt through your urine, it may also help you manage annoying pregnant bloat. Sliced bananas can be piled on top of a piece of peanut butter toast if a banana by itself isn't filling enough to serve as a snack. Alternately, put frozen banana chunks in the food processor to create a surprising amount of creamy, delectable dairy-free ice cream.

Quinoa

If you didn't consume quinoa before becoming pregnant, you should start doing so. Per cooked cup of whole grain, which is a seed, there are 8 grams of protein, 5 grams of fiber, almost 3 grams of iron, as well as trace levels of calcium, magnesium, potassium, and zinc. The best part is that quinoa cooks in under 20 minutes. For a great burrito filling, try combining it with cubes of roasted sweet potato and black beans. You can also simmer it in milk to produce a morning porridge like oatmeal.

While we're talking about the healthiest foods to consume while pregnant, keep in mind that some foods should be avoided, you should avoid certain foods until after giving birth since they are more likely to contain bacteria or chemicals that could make you ill.

Water

We must all keep ourselves hydrated. And particularly women who are pregnant. Blood volume rises by roughly 45% during pregnancy (Reliable Source). Your body will hydrate you to hydrate your unborn child, but if you don't control your water intake, you risk being dehydrated yourself. Headaches, anxiety, fatigue, a foul mood, and impaired memory are all signs of mild dehydration. Increasing your water consumption may also assist with constipation and lower your risk of urinary tract infections, which are common during pregnancy. According to general recommendations, pregnant women should consume 80 ounces (2.3 liters) of water per day. However, the precise amount you require varies. For advice tailored to your unique needs, consult your doctor.

Try keeping a reusable water bottle on hand so you can quench your thirst throughout the day. Keep in mind that you can also acquire water from other foods and beverages, such as fruit, vegetables, coffee, and tea.

The lesson

Your developing baby is eagerly anticipating nutrient-rich meals from a balanced diet of whole grains, fruits, vegetables, lean proteins, and healthy fats. You should put off doing the following for the time being:

non-pasteurized juice, untainted cheese, Fresh seafood, exotic meat.

Chapter 5

FOODS THAT DON'T FOSTER A HEALTHY PREGNANCY

Every mouthful you take in while pregnant is shared with the developing child. While some foods and even some forms of food poisoning may not damage you, they may harm your child. To prevent food poisoning, be careful not to eat any food that has been out of the refrigerator for longer than two hours (or more than one hour in hot weather). Limit your daily caffeine intake to 200 mg (one 12-ounce cup of coffee). You probably already know not to drink alcohol when you are pregnant, but you should also stay away from these foods to be safe.

Meats

Hot dogs, deli meats, cold cuts, and other prepared meats. (If heated to steaming and served hot, you can safely eat these.)

fresh, pre-stuffed turkey or chicken

Any uncooked meat, including steak tartare,

Undercooked meats and rare meat slices

Meat spreads or pates are kept in the fridge. (Meat spreads in jars and on shelves are acceptable.)

Fish

Bluefish, pike, salmon, striped bass, trout, and walleye were caught nearby.

Mercaptan-rich foods include shark, tilefish, swordfish, and king mackerel. Smoked cod, smoked lox, smoked trout, smoked tuna, smoked whitefish, or any other smoked fish

Sushi, raw fish, or raw shellfish of any kind (oysters, clams, mussels)

Eggs

A raw egg

Uncooked cookie dough (It contains raw eggs.) Mayonnaise, bearnaise, hollandaise, Caesar salad dressing, and any other homemade dressings and sauces created using raw eggs. Any homemade delicacies prepared with raw eggs, such as mousse, meringue, tiramisu, etc.

Cheese and Milk (untainted milk)

any cheese produced from raw milk. Soft cheeses like Brie, blue cheese, feta, panela, queso Blanco, and queso fresco are more likely to be manufactured from raw milk than hard cheeses. However, certain raw milk cheeses are available in the United States; always check the labels.

Veggies and fruits

fresh juice purchased from a store or any unpasteurized juice, Fresh produce that hasn't been washed, Fresh sprouts, Unripe papaya.

Chapter 6

EXPECTATIONS FOR PREGNANCY AND COMMON COMPLAINTS

A woman's body goes through various changes while she is pregnant. The majority of frequent symptoms are natural and typically result from changes in your body, including as the growth of your uterus and unborn child, as well as the volume and fluid content of your blood. But how can you tell if your problem is typical or needs more investigation? Common concerns are not usually indicative of normal behavior. Most of the complaints during pregnancy includes:

Daytime sickness

In the first trimester of pregnancy, nausea and sickness are particularly frequent. Although it is commonly experienced during the first three months of pregnancy, morning sickness can linger for the entire day and may even last longer for some people. Most patients will have nausea but may not become unwell, while other women may find they are unable to swallow any food. Hormones that aid in the growth of the fetus and placenta are what induce morning sickness. Although the symptoms are uncomfortable, the developing baby won't be harmed by them. Morning sickness can be avoided by:

Taking frequent, little meals, consuming dry, carbohydrate nibbles all day long.

Taking breaks during the day, drinking plenty of water, and avoiding alcohol and coffee. Don't wear restrictive apparel; it will just make you feel worse.

Inform your midwife or doctor if you are always unwell and unable to swallow meals. Some pregnant women have quite bad nausea and vomiting. Hyperemesis gravidarum is the medical term for this disorder, which requires specialized care.

Constipation

Early in pregnancy, because of the hormonal changes occurring in your body, you could experience constipation. Constipation can be avoided by; consuming fiber-rich foods such as wholemeal bread, wholegrain cereals, fruit, vegetables, beans, and lentils.

Regular exercise will help you maintain muscle tone.

Consuming a lot of water

Avoid taking iron supplements; instead, consult your physician to see if you can get by without them or switch to a different kind.

Treatment of pregnancy pain

Women who are pregnant may experience moderate headaches and other aches and pains. Non-steroidal anti-inflammatory medicines (NSAIDs), such as ibuprofen(external link opens in a new window/tab), should not be used during pregnancy. This is true of several painkillers. They might impede kidney function, induce early labor, or cause miscarriage in the early stages. Since it can raise the risk of bleeding, aspirin is not advised for pain treatment. Codeine-based analgesics should only be used in the early stages of pregnancy under a doctor's supervision because they can create respiratory issues for the unborn child in the later stages. Although paracetamol is safe, it should only be used during pregnancy if required and for the smallest amount of time. Before using any OTC medication, if you get sick with a cold while pregnant, be sure to talk to your pharmacist. Many will include Codeine or antihistamines, which are not recommended during pregnancy. Paracetamol will ease headaches.

Skin changes

During pregnancy, many women will notice changes in their skin. The majority of these alterations are classified as "physiological," which denotes that they are completely normal and connected to pregnancy. Darkening of the nipples and vaginal region is known as hyperpigmentation. Linea Nigra – a dark, sometimes hairy, line that runs from the belly button to the pubic area. Stretch marks known as striae gravidarum appear on the belly as it swells; they typically start pink and turn white or shiny after delivery. Legs with varicose veins

Rashes

Rashes like eczema and psoriasis can also be problematic for expectant mothers. You might ask your doctor whether it's safe and recommended to use steroid cream or another type of lotion.

In addition,

Pregnancy-specific rashes are known as particular dermatoses (skin diseases). Generalized rashes that can happen at any time without a rash, itching. These disorders can cause harm to mother and baby, so seek medical advice if you spot skin changes that seem abnormal. Itching without a rash during pregnancy can be normal or problematic. If you have itching, especially if it keeps growing worse, you should get advice.

Ankles, feet, and finger swelling

Because your body is storing more water than usual during pregnancy, your fingers, ankles, and feet may occasionally swell somewhat.

Swelling can be reduced by:

avoiding prolonged standing putting on cozy shoes. Whenever you can recline your chair

working out your feet. Ask your doctor or midwife to check your blood pressure if the swelling does not go down.

Gums and teeth

You should visit your dentist for a checkup because dental care is free during pregnancy and for a year following the birth of your child. Pregnancy should always be disclosed to your dentist as it may influence your care.

Your gums may become more irritated, swollen, and prone to bleeding due to hormonal changes that occur during pregnancy. Your gums should return to normal once your baby is born. Consult with your dentist to determine whether any new or replacement fillings need to wait until the baby is delivered.

Dilated veins

Veins that swell up are referred to as varicose veins. Inform your doctor if you suffer from varicose veins or if a close family has ever experienced a blood clot or clotting disease. If you have vein problems; avoiding prolonged standing. Avoid sitting with your legs crossed. Avoid gaining too much weight. To reduce pain, raise your legs when you are sitting. Test out support tights. When you sleep, elevate your legs above your body. Try antenatal exercise to improve your blood flow.

Virulent discharge

Pregnancy increases vaginal discharge for almost all women. It ought to be white and transparent, and it shouldn't smell bad. You can have an infection if your discharge is colored, smells unusual, or causes you to feel itchy or sore.

Thrush is the most typical infection, and your doctor can readily treat it. Wearing undergarments made of loose cotton can help avoid thrush.

Heartburn

Your heart has nothing to do with heartburn. It is a digestive issue. Sometimes heartburn is referred to as acid indigestion or acid reflux. You may have a sharp burning pain beneath your breastbone or ribs (around your heart), anywhere along the passageway from the back of your throat to your stomach, when digestive acids leak out of the stomach. It is brought on by the stress of the developing baby and variations in hormone levels during pregnancy.

To feel better, try this. After eating, avoid lying down. When you do lie down, raise your head and shoulders Avoid fried or greasy foods. Drink fluids between meals, instead of with your meal. Avoid coffee, colas, alcohol, and smoking. Eat slowly and chew your food well. Eat small meals and snacks rather than a huge meal at once.

When to see your care provider

Very important: Some women take an antacid pill to aid with heartburn. An antacid decreases the amount of acid in your stomach. Antacids are not all safe for expectant mothers to take. Before you take one, consult your healthcare provider.

Nausea and diarrhea

Even though nausea and vomiting can occur at any time of day, many women experience them frequently. Hormone changes can make you feel queasy, especially during the first three months of pregnancy. The good news is that this daily queasy feeling typically goes away by the fourth month of your pregnancy.

To feel better, try this; Avoid going to bed hungry. Eat whatever you frequently want in small amounts until you feel better. Slowly get out of bed and then have breakfast. Instead of doing so while you're eating, drink fluids between meals. If possible, choose cold foods (which have less smell) or have someone else cook for you.

Take in a lot of fresh air. Take in the aroma of freshly cut lemons. Avoid alcohol, coffee, strong odors, and smoking.

Swelling

In the third trimester, many women have mild swelling or edema in their feet and ankles. Pregnancy hormones cause women to naturally retain more water in their bodies; thus, this is normal, even if it can be very painful. Alternatively, they can feel puffy or bloated throughout their pregnancy. The day after your baby is born, it will disappear. Even when you feel bloated, it's crucial to keep drinking water and other liquids to be healthy.

To feel better, try this; Raise your feet

Do not cross your legs. Don comfortable clothing and shoes. Get lots of rest and activity.

Important: While you are pregnant, avoid using water pills or over-the-counter or herbal diuretics. Consult your healthcare practitioner.

How often should you visit your doctor?

A more serious ailment may show symptoms of certain forms of edema. As soon as you see any of the following: Any facial or hand edema that is more than a little severe. Any sudden, painful, or swollen ankles or feet, an intractable headache. Vision changes like sensitivity to light or blurry vision. Uneven swelling, when one ankle is larger than the other, etc. Painful swelling of any kind

Chapter 7

MEAL PLANS

Meal planning can help you eat a wider range of meals and more fruits and vegetables, which can lower your chance of developing chronic lifestyle diseases. You can help guarantee that you're eating the appropriate foods in the right amounts by creating a healthy meal plan to ensure you're getting plenty of nutrients.

What kind of diet is ideal for expectant mothers?

Vegetables, fruits, proteins, whole grains, and a variety of meals are all part of a healthy pregnancy meal plan for women who are expecting. This ensures that you and your unborn child get all the nutrients you need. Keep in touch with your doctor and pay attention to your body throughout each trimester. Depending on how you're feeling, each stage can call for a varied calorie intake.

What can I eat for breakfast, lunch, and dinner when I'm pregnant?

In addition to whole grains and water, a pregnant woman should try to eat protein, fruit, and vegetables at most meals. You may get the nutrients you and your baby need to feel strong and healthy by consuming a variety of meals. It is recommended that pregnant women consume at least eight glasses of water each day.

Healthy breakfasts during pregnancy:

Nonfat Greek yogurt with berries, chia seeds, flax seeds, and honey. Smoothies made with yogurt, fruits, vegetables, and protein powder. Egg quiche without a crust, such as this or this Served with a side of bacon or turkey sausage, hard-boiled eggs

Steel-cut oats with milk, berries, almonds, and raisins on top. Eggs with toast and fruit on the side. sandwiches made with bagels

pancakes with protein and peanut butter. pregnancy-friendly lunches. Wrapped chicken salad, sprinkled with cinnamon and baked sweet potatoes. Cucumber salad with quinoa, potatoes baked in a cheese and broccoli sauce, the turkey burger.

Sandwich with tuna, zucchini burgers, Bean soup, meal leftovers

Thai coconut curry with chicken

Salad of broccoli

healthy meals for pregnant women

like this or this stir-fry

Enchiladas, fajitas, or tacos

cabbage stuffed

sandwiches with chopped chicken

Such bean or chicken burrito bowls

baked chicken breast and vegetables on the side

Chicken-flavored ravioli or tortellini

Greek chicken with lemon and potatoes

Lentils and shrimp from India

Fish like this salmon or this perch, but keep in mind that the recommended weekly serving size for pregnant women is 12 ounces of fish.

Chops of pork and veggies

Zucchini with Italian sausage filling

Grilled chicken from Asia

Suitable snack options

Edamame

Smoothie

Cheese in slices

Nuts \Berries

Vegetables with hummus or a dressing

Energy spheres

Banana or apple and peanut butter

Cheese cottage

Greek yogurt portions

Toast spread with almond or peanut butter

Milk and a bowl of cereal or granola

anything from the breakfast selections

Ideas for healthy treats

Energy spheres

a chocolate bar

A serving of ice cream

Oatmeal raisin cookies

Italian lemon ice-cream sherbet

Raspberry crumble

Banana bread slice

A Sample Pregnancy Menu

Here is an example of a daily menu created especially for our "sample mom," along with a few more snack ideas. Although your menu may resemble this one, you may get a personalized plan by registering at ChooseMyPlate.gov.

Breakfast

Cantaloupe, half a cup

Using one teaspoon of canola oil, scramble two eggs with 1/4 cup each of bell pepper and mushrooms.

a single whole wheat bread piece with a single teaspoon of butter

one cup of nonfat milk

Snack

a single big apple

Lunch

3/4 cup chili with beans and two tablespoons grated cheddar cheese are placed on top of one medium baked potato.

Two tablespoons of light salad dressing and one tablespoon of dried cranberries added to 1 cup of spinach salad

Two crackers made of rye crispbread

one cup of nonfat milk

Snack

Baby carrots, 1/2 cup

3 cups of air-popped corn (includes one teaspoon of oil)

Advertisement | Below is a further page

Dinner

Four ounces of grilled salmon with 1/2 a sliced tomato and 1/4 a sliced avocado.

1 cup cooked quinoa or brown rice

12 cup cooked green beans

one roll of whole grain

Orange Snack, one

Milk, low-fat, 8 ounces

little oatmeal cookies

This typical daily menu contains 3 1/4 cups of vegetables, slightly more than 2 cups of fruit, 8 ounces of meat and beans, 7 ounces of grains, 3 1/3 cups of dairy products, and two tablespoons of healthy fats and oils for a total of little less than 2,200 calories.

Chapter 8

EXERCISE

How much exercise is necessary while pregnant?

At least 212 hours of moderate-intensity aerobic activity are required each week for healthy pregnant women. Exercises that involve an aerobic component cause your heart rate and breathing rate to increase. You are sufficiently active at a moderate intensity to perspire and raise your heart rate. A quick walk is an illustration of moderate-intensity aerobic exercise. If you find it difficult to speak normally while working out, you might be working too hard.

Not all 2 12 hours have to be completed at once. Instead, divide it up over the week. Do 30 minutes of exercise, for instance, most days or always. If 30 minutes seems excessive, break it up into three 10-minute sessions of exercise each day.

What types of activities are safe to engage in while pregnant?

It's usually safe to continue your activities during pregnancy if you're healthy and were an active person before becoming pregnant. To be certain, confirm with your provider. For example, if you're a runner or a tennis player or you do other kinds of intense exercise, you may be able to keep doing your workouts when you're pregnant. As your belly gets bigger later in pregnancy, you may need to change some activities or ease up on your workouts.

If your provider says it's OK for you to exercise, choose activities you enjoy. If you didn't exercise before you were pregnant, now is a great time to start. Talk to your provider about safe activities. Start slowly and build up your fitness little by little. For example, start with 5 minutes of activity each day, and work your way up to 30 minutes each day.

These activities normally are safe during pregnancy:

Walking:

A fast walk is an excellent exercise that is gentle on your joints and muscles. This is a fantastic workout to get started with.

Swimming and water exercises:

The weight of your growing baby is supported by the water, and working out in the water helps raise your heart rate. It's also gentle on your muscles and joints. Try swimming if you experience low back pain during other activities.

Cycling on a stationary bike is safer during pregnancy than cycling on a conventional bicycle. Even as your belly swells, you're less likely to fall off a stationary bike than on a conventional bike.

Inform your yoga or Pilates instructor what you are expecting during a lesson.

The instructor can assist you in modifying or avoiding poses, like as reclining on your stomach or lying flat on your back, that might be harmful to expectant women (after the first trimester). Only for pregnant women, some gyms and community centers offer prenatal yoga and Pilates programs.

Low-impact aerobics classes:

You always have one foot on the ground or equipment during low-impact aerobics. Walking, utilizing an elliptical machine, and stationary biking are a few examples of low-impact aerobics. Your body won't be as taxed by low-impact aerobics as it will be by high-impact aerobics. In high-impact aerobics, both feet lift off the floor simultaneously. Running, jumping rope, and jumping jacks are a few examples. Informing your trainer of your pregnancy will enable them to assist you in modifying your workout as necessary.

Strength training:

Strength training can help you increase your muscle mass and strengthen your bones. Weightlifting is safe as long as the weights are not excessive. Inquire with your provider about your lifting capacity. To be active, you don't need to own specialized equipment or subscribe to a gym. You can watch fitness videos at home or go for a walk in a secure area. Or look for methods to be more active every day, such as working in the yard or choosing the stairs over the elevator.

Why is exercise healthy for a pregnant woman?

For pregnant women in good health, regular exercise can:

1. Keep your body and mind in good shape. You can feel better and have more energy by engaging in physical activity. Additionally, it strengthens your blood vessels, heart, and lungs while keeping you physically healthy.

2. assist you in gaining the appropriate amount of weight while pregnant.

3. reduce some of the usual pregnant discomforts, including back pain, swelling in the legs, ankles, and feet, and constipation.

4. aid in better sleep and stress management. Stress is anxiety, strain, or pressure that you experience as a result of events in your life.

5. lower your risk of developing preeclampsia and gestational diabetes throughout pregnancy. One type of diabetes

that can develop during pregnancy is gestational diabetes. It takes place when your blood has an excessive amount of glucose or sugar. Preeclampsia is a form of high blood pressure that some pregnant women have after the 20th week or immediately following delivery. These disorders can raise your chance of pregnancy difficulties, such as an early birth (birth before 37 weeks of pregnancy).

6. assist in lowering the risk of giving birth via c-section (also called c-section). Cesarean delivery is a surgical procedure in which your doctor creates a cut in your abdomen and uterus to deliver your baby.

7. Get your body ready for labor and delivery. You can practice breathing, meditation, and other relaxing techniques

that may help you manage labor pain through exercises like prenatal yoga and Pilates. Regular exercise can help you have the power and energy you need during birth.

Which workouts ought to be avoided when pregnant?

There are some exercises and activities that should not be done while pregnant. Avoid:

- Staying still while engaging in any activity

- Activities that put you at risk of falling (such as skiing and horseback riding)

- Contact sports like basketball, volleyball, football, and softball

- Any exercise that could result in even minor abdominal stress, such as jarring motions or sudden changes in direction

- Activities that call for a lot of hopping, skipping, jumping, or bouncing

- Deep knee bends, complete sit-ups, double leg lifts, and toe touches with a straight leg

- Bouncing and extending